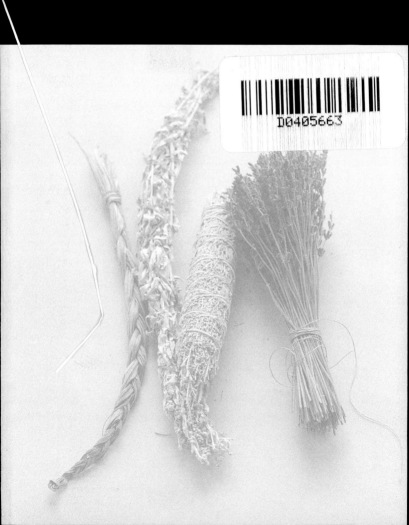

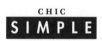

CHIC
SIMPLE
Components

"The sense of smell is the sense of imagination."

JEAN-JACQUES ROUSSEAU

CHIC

SIMPLE

Components

S C E N T S

ALFRED A. KNOPF   NEW YORK 1993

THIS IS A BORZOI BOOK
PUBLISHED BY ALFRED A. KNOPF, INC.

KIM JOHNSON GROSS   JEFF STONE

WRITTEN BY JANINE KING
PHOTOGRAPHS BY MARIA ROBLEDO
ICON ILLUSTRATION BY ERIC HANSEN
RESEARCHED BY KIMBERLY PASQUALE
STYLED BY HANNAH MILMAN

DESIGN AND ART DIRECTION BY ROBERT VALENTINE
INCORPORATED

Library of Congress Cataloging-in-Publication Data
Gross, Kim Johnson.
Chic simple. Scents / Kim Johnson Gross, Jeff Stone, and Janine King.
p. cm.—(Chic simple)
ISBN 0-679-42764-3
1. Perfumes. 2. Potpourris (Scented floral mixtures). 3. Odors.
I. Stone, Jeff. II. King, Janine. III. Title. IV. Title: Scents. V. Series.
GT2340.G77 1993
391'.63—dc20
93-20309
CIP

Manufactured in the United States of America
First Edition

CONTENTS

SCENTS
*The historical and physiological appreciation
of scent*
11

ELEMENTS
Herbs, citrus, flowers, woods, spices
31

DIFFUSION
Ways to bring scent home
57

FIRST AID
*Tips to hold fresh, balanced, lasting fragrances
in the home*
80

WHERE
*Worldwide guide to environmental-scent sources,
outlets, and catalogues*
83

"The more you know, the less you need."

AUSTRALIAN ABORIGINAL SAYING

Chic Simple is a primer for living well but sensibly in the 1990s. It's for those who believe that quality of life does not come in accumulating things, but in paring down to the essentials, with a commitment to home, community, and the environment. In a world of limited resources, Chic Simple enables readers to bring value and style into their lives with economy and simplicity.

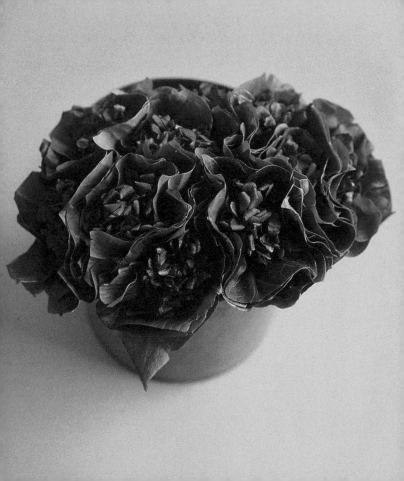

S C E N T S

A scent can be the hint of a past or a promise. It is the touch of an airborne molecule to the most primal of all animal senses, a key to one of the millions of olfactory receptor-locks, a message to the brain—of sustenance, calm, excitement, danger. Through the ageless art of scent, fragrance works its desired effect on the psyche.

"Smells are surer than sounds and sights to
make the heartstrings crack."

RUDYARD KIPLING

HISTORY OF THE SCENT.

EXPRESSION BY SCENT—OR REPRESSION OF SMELL, as Freud put it—has always been a universal sign of civilization. Since ancient Egypt, perfumes have sweetened the body and soul, the skin and the temple. Fresh and dried aromatics were always appreciated, but with the tenth-century discovery of oil distillation, the most fleeting fragrance was captured for commerce. The perfume trades seized—and ultimately synthesized—all earthly scents, from the simple sweetness of a violet to the complexity of a breeze. Today, most products, even the "unscented," are dashed with fragrance.

SCENTS OF THE GREAT

Queen of Sheba: myrrh
Queen Hatshepsut: cedar
Nero: rose
Mohammed: musk
Indra: jasmine
Louis XIV: orange/clove
Napoleon: rosemary
Josephine: violets
Montezuma: cocoa/vanilla
Chanel: #5

ENDLESS SCENT

Musk, the most tenacious scent, is still detected in one-thousand-year-old mosques constructed with perfumed mortar that exude scent when heated by the sun. Also, despite repaintings, musk lingers at Malmaison, which the Empress Josephine perfumed lavishly.

The American Museum of Natural History enhances its habitat displays
with synthesized scents.

Fragrance systems are often installed in Japanese office buildings; rosemary
and lemon piped through work areas increase productivity, and jasmine
and chamomile help employees relax in lounge and dining rooms.

Environmental officials in Munich are developing an odor map of the city
to diagnose and eliminate problem smells.

"The past is the only dead thing that smells sweet."

EDWARD THOMAS

TIME SCENTS

B.C. Geishas to the court of Japan were paid by the number of fifteen-
minute incense sticks burned.

A.D. Seiko has introduced a "fragrance alarm clock" that releases a
stimulating eucalyptus-and-pine scent before the beeper sounds.

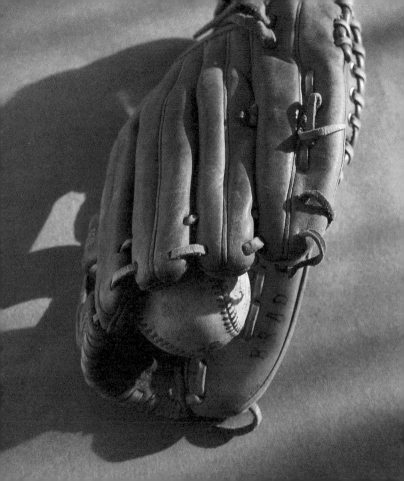

Scent Memory. Scent can bring back a moment in time with startling clarity. Unlike the other senses, smell channels directly to the brain's limbic system, home to memory, emotion, and imagination. Memory mysteriously holds scent in ways that defy logic, for scents are neither isolated nor pure (coffee, for instance, includes over 400 scent variables). A whiff of leather can conjure up a wide range of associations— a baseball mitt, a shoe, a Filofax, a new car—or it can inexplicably evoke some exotic and reckless moment with perfect precision. But some associations are more abstract: "The scent of bitter almonds always reminded him of the fate of unrequited love," Gabriel García Márquez wrote of the telltale sign of cyanide in *Love in the Time of Cholera*.

SO GOES THE NOSE

Do the senses of smell and memory grow in tandem? The sense of smell is keenest at middle age, and, as indicated from studies of Alzheimer's patients, the faculties of smell and memory fade together.

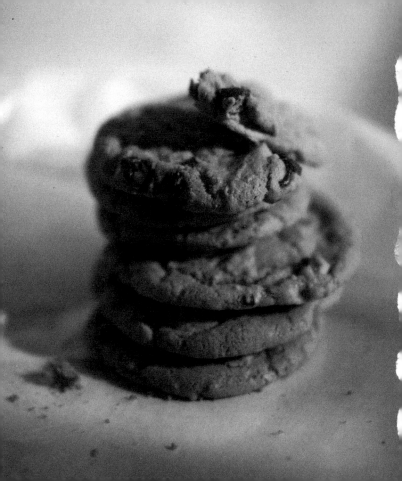

Scent and Taste. Nature made the nose for sniffing out edibles—for distinguishing the foul from the fresh. Without smell, there are no flavors and only four taste distinctions—sweet, sour, bitter, and salty; without smell, there's no telling an apple from an onion. Because appetite, like memory, emotion, and smell, is centered in the limbic system, adults strongly associate food with childhood. However, young children do not naturally scent-discriminate and must learn what smells "good" and "bad." The emotional response to scents is not universal, but rather a matter of experience.

BREAKFAST
A pellet releases the smell of bagels when heated by the neon-sign displays of Seattle's Spot Bagel Bakery.

APPLE A DAY
The scent of apples is comforting, a point noted by Queen Mary Tudor's physician in the sixteenth century and confirmed by recent Yale studies.

MUNCHIES
Guy de Maupassant needed the scent of strawberries to work.

TAKEOUT
The diets of Indians and Thais make their bodies smell good; the Japanese diet accounts for little body odor. Foods affect how the body smells for more than twenty-four hours.

Scents of Well-Being. The average person can detect about 10,000 scents, not all of them agreeable. Some people neutralize their environments by opening and closing windows, while others disguise odors by a diffusion of pleasing scents. True scent enthusiasts manage fragrance to its full psyche-soothing or stimulating powers. Science confirms that certain scents can have therapeutic benefit to the respiratory system, and can alter mood, alertness, and productivity. A link between personal fragrance and social interaction (particularly between people of opposite sex) is also established. The practice of aromatherapy expands on these notions.

SAFETY SCENTS
General Motors is exploring automobile fragrance systems to keep drivers attentive.

IN-SCENTIVES
A study showed that people were more likely to buy Nike shoes in a scented environment, and to gamble in scented casinos.

SCENT NOT
Researchers at Johns Hopkins are seeking scent "antagonists," molecules that would block foul smells, which might be sprayed in restrooms.

SMELL-A-VISION
During Hollywood's fling with scented movies, the audience was exposed to odors matched to screen images.

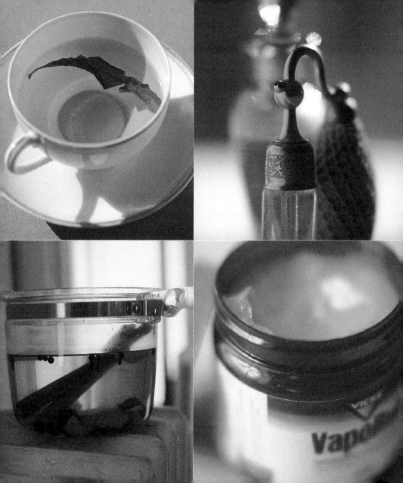

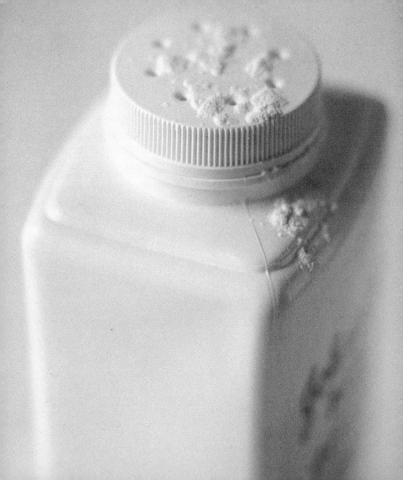

Simple Scents. Everyone has a personal scent, unique as a fingerprint. It is not just a matter of hygiene, but also of diet, hormones, health, coloring, age, variations in mood and temperature, and, many scientists believe, subliminal scent-beams of desire called pheromones. To a loved one, the body aroma is both recognizable and alluring; mothers and newborns will respond to each other's scent within two days. To strangers, it may be as unattractive as Madison Avenue says; anthropologist Margaret Mead found a tribe so antagonized by another's scent that they waged war. The simplest scent is of self.

SCENT-YES
Elizabethan women offered "love apples" imbued with their underarm sweat to ardent suitors.

SCENT-LESS
Excessive body odor has been cause for rejection from military service in Japan.

SCENT-SIMPLE
The scent of Johnson's baby powder—recognized as simplicity itself—is a closely guarded secret blend of 262 ingredients.

SCENT-MORE
Women have a keener sense of smell than men, and their acuity intensifies at ovulation.

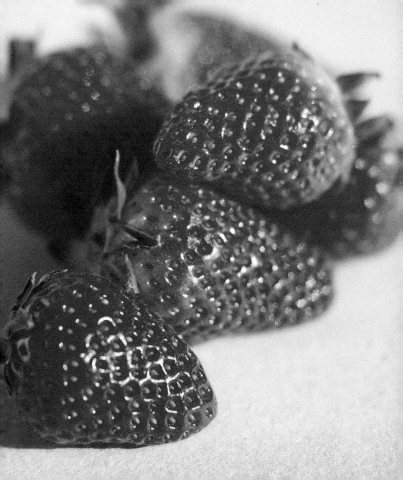

Seduction. Throughout the ages, perfumers and their clientele have struggled in vain to find the surefire aphrodisiac. When asked to grade the importance of smell in sexual relationships on a scale of 1 to 10, women responded 8.5 and men 7.5. Women are attracted by potent scents such as jasmine and, especially, musk, which resembles testosterone and is detectable in infinitesimal amounts (although many men and children do not smell musk at all). Men are aroused by clean scents like lavender, rosemary, and cedar, as well as the subliminally recognized scents of ovulating women and, curiously, redheads.

HIDE AND GO SCENT
Madame de Pompadour fixed tiny individually scented star and crescent patches all over her body for the King to delight in finding.

"Only the nose knows where the nose goes when the door close."
MUHAMMAD ALI

PASSION SCENT
Cleopatra first met Mark Antony on her royal barge whose purple sails were drenched in perfume.

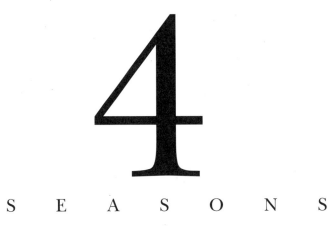

SEASONS

Abundant, organic, and freely relished without any intervention by man, the scents of nature are a simple pleasure of great chemical complexity. The fragrant molecules of plants, the "essential oils," are by-products of metabolism to satisfy needs for protection or pollination. But the perfume of the outdoors includes the smells of beached seaweed, earth freshly turned with manure, burning leaves, and all the other residues of the living that add a pungency appreciable only in the wild.

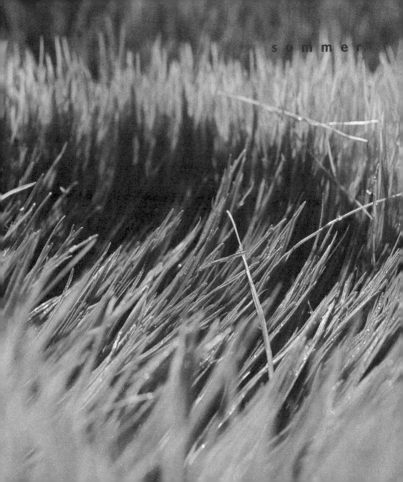

summer

Evergreens are nature's own antidepressants, which explains the ancient widespread custom of bringing freshly cut, fragrant boughs into the home during the bleak winter months.

The sweetness of spring's new growth and autumn's initial decay can be alike chemically; the scents of narcissus and lilac, for instance, include alcohol indol, a product of decomposition.

spring and fall

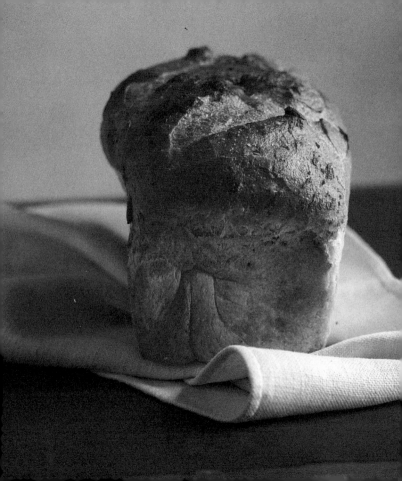

interiors

THE ARCHITECTURAL EQUIVALENT OF ONE'S
UNIQUE BODY SCENT IS THE SMELL OF ONE'S HOME,
COMFORTING TO THOSE WHO ARE ACCUSTOMED TO IT AND
curious to outsiders. Here are the smells of the stove and refrigerator, laundry freshly spun in the dryer or still soiled in the
basket, puppy fur, and wood polish. People who actively scent
their interiors introduce outdoor fragrances to the indoor
bouquet. Some travel with a vial of their preferred scent to
remind them of home, but it falls short of the truth; the complex aroma of a home is inimitable. Nothing else smells like home.

SCENTS OF COMFORT *The smell of fresh-baked bread is so reminiscent*
of the happiness of home that it has been re-created in room sprays to help sell
real estate. There are also "new-car" scented sprays to help sell old jalopies.

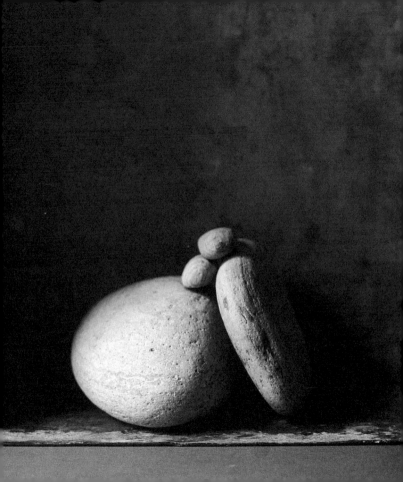

ELEMENTS

Since ancient times, nature's most aromatic treasures have been gathered into a dark cool place for drying, distilling, blending, and preserving. This fragrant way station to perfumes and flavorings was called "the still room" in medieval Europe, a name that remains in use today.

"A perfume is more than an extraction: it is a presence in abstraction."

GIORGIO ARMANI

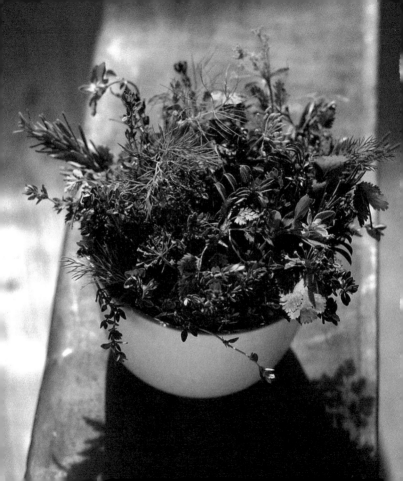

Aromatic Herbs. The fresh aroma of the herbal bouquet ranges from sweet to camphoric. Usually invigorating, herbs can smell faintly medicinal and have a long history of pharmaceutical use. Both fresh and dry herbs hold their fragrance for extended periods, none more so than rosemary. Strongly antiseptic and purifying, rosemary has been burned as incense, strewn on the floors of homes, carried in antiplague nosegays, placed in drawers to repel moths, tucked into potpourri, sachets, and pillows. Rosemary is widely used in perfume products, most notably in cologne and men's aftershave.

ENTICING
Rosemary was an ingredient in "Hungary Water," the first alcoholic perfume, created in the fourteenth century especially for the aged Queen of Hungary to help her catch a new husband.

REPELLENT
Mint deters mice, rosemary repels moths and garden pests, catnip keeps ants and beetles away.

OVERLOAD
The cleanup crew of a coriander spill at an herb distillery became giggly, then violent, then nauseated and had to be sent home to recover.

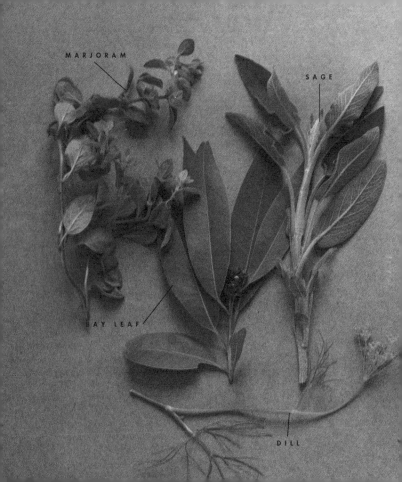

MARJORAM

SAGE

BAY LEAF

DILL

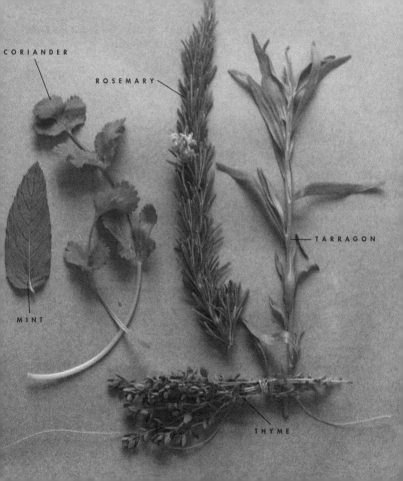

CORIANDER

ROSEMARY

MINT

TARRAGON

THYME

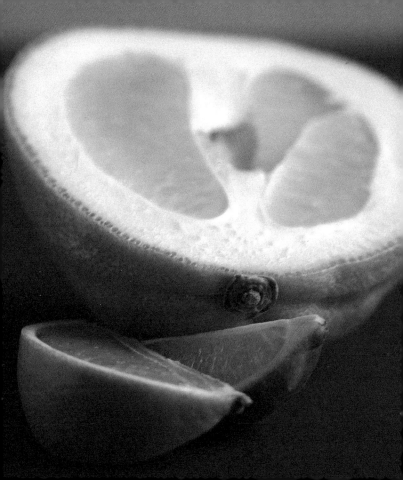

Citrus. The sweetly astringent scent of the citrus family evokes a feeling of cleanliness that has brought it to a prominent position in perfuming products as diverse as today's furniture polish and yesteryear's colognes. The essence of citrus blossom is the delicate neroli oil, among the most precious scents in the perfumer's kit. Petitgrain is the oil extracted from orange leaves and twigs. Other scents, including bergamot, mandarin, orange, lemon, and lime, are derived from pressed rind. Some botanicals, such as lemon verbena, share the chemistry of citrus scent and often take on its role in perfumes, soaps, and flavorings.

SCENT APPEAL
Citrus perfume appeals to extroverts.

SCENTS PER POUND
One ton of citrus blossoms yields just two pounds of neroli oil.

SCENT IMMACULATE
The sweet-orange groves of Mediterranean Europe are the progeny of a single tree, still preserved in Lisbon, that Vasco da Gama brought back from China.

NEW SCENTS
Columbus brought the first orange trees to America.

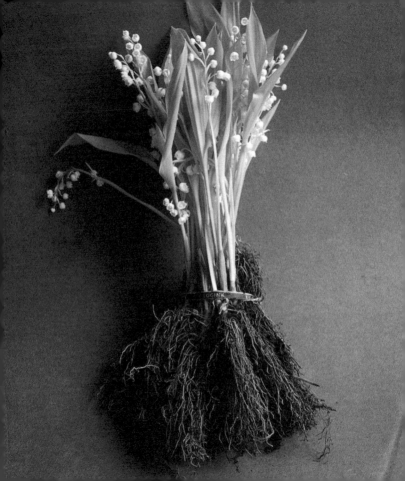

Floral. Flowers possess Nature's most complex scents in terms of chemistry, and they also elicit the strongest emotional response. They are flirtatious or cheerful or deeply intoxicating to the point of provocation. While the scents of greens and wood were meant to repel predators, nature designed floral scents to entice pollinators. White flowers are usually the most fragrant. Their fragrance and their sheen in moonlight woo the night-flying numb-nosed moth rather than the nimbler bees and butterflies, which service the reds, pinks, and yellows. White flowers are the heart and soul of perfumery.

WE AND THE BEE
Smell acuity and preferences are similar in humans and honeybees. By contrast, a dog's sense of smell is forty-four times stronger and favors odors that are disagreeable to man and bee.

MOONLIGHTING
10,600 jasmine blossoms and twenty-eight dozen roses, all picked by hand before dawn, go into a single ounce of Joy from Patou.

WHITE MISCHIEF
The lily of the valley defies bottling: for perfume, its scent is re-created by aroma chemicals laced with ylang-ylang, orange blossom, jasmine, and rose oil.

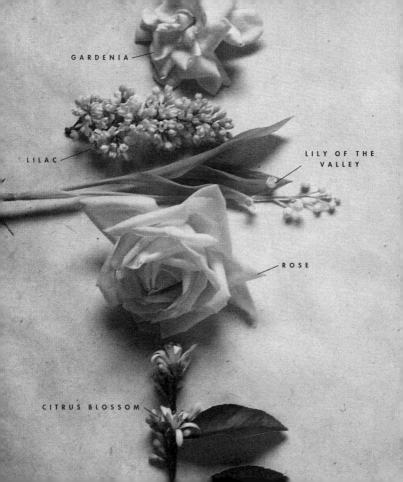

GARDENIA

LILAC

LILY OF THE
VALLEY

ROSE

CITRUS BLOSSOM

TUBEROSE

FREESIA

JASMINE

HYACINTH

ROSEBUD

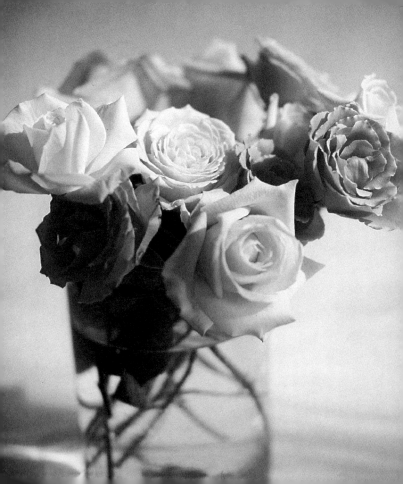

Roses. Roses are more antiseptic than citrus and higher in vitamin C. Until the nineteenth century, they figured in more than one-third of all remedies for ailments, from depression to infertility, and were the leading sweetener of food. They are the star of mythology, the blood of Venus, the sweat of Mohammed, a secret of Coca-Cola. Roses were the passion of Romans who bathed in them, slept on them, and dropped them by the net loads over orgies (sweetly suffocating one guest, it is recorded). They are of such delicate beauty and scent that poets swoon, but so hardy that they can withstand the heat of the distillery. Roses ramble through every garden, but reign from one 80-by-30-mile patch of damask rose on a Bulgarian mountaintop where drop by precious tiny drop per thirty hand-plucked blossoms, they yield the perfumer's oil. The rose is exceptional, the all-time favorite flower.

"Rose is a rose is a rose is a rose."

GERTRUDE STEIN, *Sacred Emily*

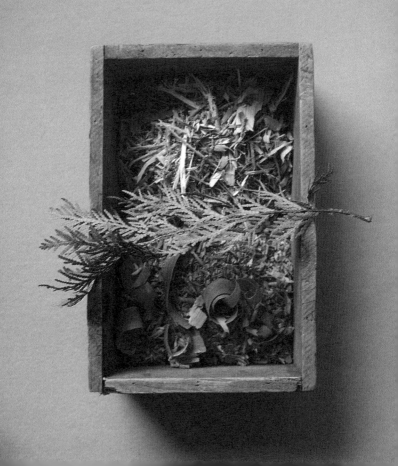

Woodland. The smells of the heartwood and their resins, of the needles, and of the forest floor may be deep and dusky or they may strike the nose with a high-pitched tingle. Either way, they tend to evoke profound spiritual or meditative response, for these were the first aromas to please man and his gods. These are the smells of religion.

"You drink the scent of the woods like water from the spring."

CHANG CHEN, A.D. 725

CEDAR
Civilizations have revered cedar for its preservative and insect-repellent properties.

ANCIENT CEDAR
Egyptians fought wars to secure its supply for the doors of tombs and for use in embalming.

AMERICAN CEDAR
North American plainsmen hung western cedar from their tepee tops, believing that it discouraged lightning as well as pests.

CEDAR WISDOM
Cedar, fir, and pine are soothing; cypress and juniper are energizing.

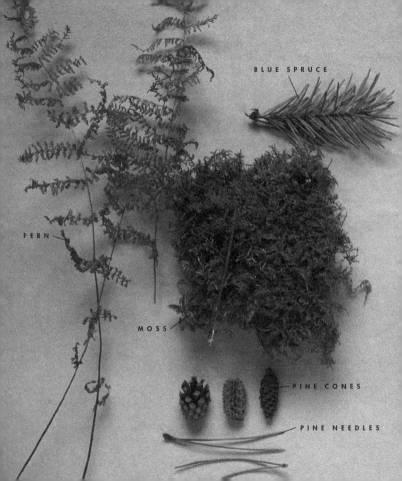

BLUE SPRUCE

FERN

MOSS

PINE CONES

PINE NEEDLES

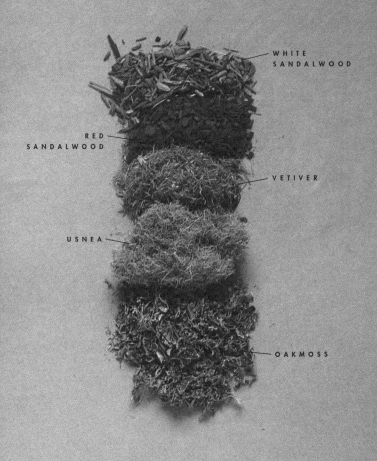

WHITE
SANDALWOOD

RED
SANDALWOOD

VETIVER

USNEA

OAKMOSS

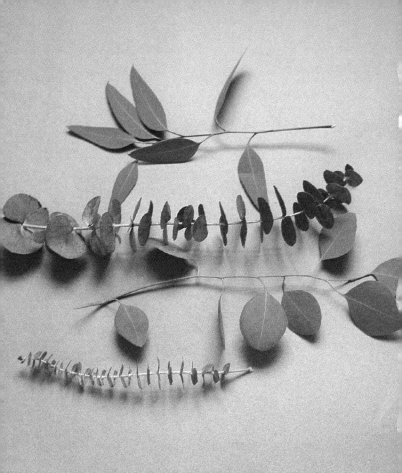

Therapeutic. Some woodland scents have therapeutic value whether in the form of drops of essential oil on a hankie or fresh branches hung in a steamy shower. Scottish Highlanders burned stubs of pine root to sweeten their cottages. The aromas of the conifer family—particularly pine, fir, and spruce—are tonic and appeasing to the nervous and respiratory systems, as well as aiding the spirit. Eucalyptus is even more potent. This native of Australia, where it was considered a cure-all by the aborigines, is today widely prescribed for conditions such as flu, asthma, cough, and bronchitis.

KNOCK ON WOOD
The phrase "keeping at bay" derives from the ancient belief that bay leaves deter plague and evil spirits.

HARDWOOD
Sandalwood has a long history in Eastern medicine and is still used in Ayurveda, the ancient Indian practice of holistic medicine; the scent is relaxing, antidepressant, and, some say, an aphrodisiac.

WOOD OHM
Blue spruce is recommended for yoga, meditation, and "psychic work."

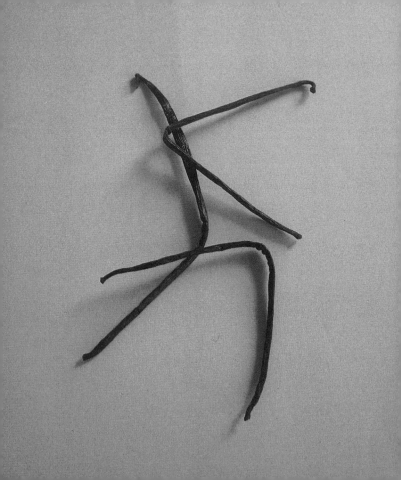

Spices. The scent of spice is warm, uplifting, piquant, sometimes exotic, sometimes homey, and always redolent of the aromas of fine cuisine. Of all the spices, cinnamon has been the most universally coveted. This curly snap of Nepalese bark has spiked the medications of the Chinese Emperor Shen Nung, the perfumes of Cleopatra, and the breakfast buns of Sara Lee. Cinnamon was the goal of the sixteenth-century European race around the Cape of Good Hope to the East Indies spice islands. But the vanilla bean, an American native, was sweet consolation to westward explorers, for, after saffron, vanilla has been the most expensive of spices.

VANILLA FACT
Vanilla is the only orchid used in perfumery.

VANILLA EXTRACT
Madagascar is today's leading producer of true vanilla.

PLASTIC VANILLA
The Ontario Paper Company is the leading producer of synthetic vanilla, which is derived from by-products of paper manufacturing or coal tar.

VANILLA PEACE
Vanilla scent has relaxed patients undergoing MRI scans at Sloan Kettering Cancer Center.

ANGELICA

CINNAMON

CARDAMOM

LICORICE

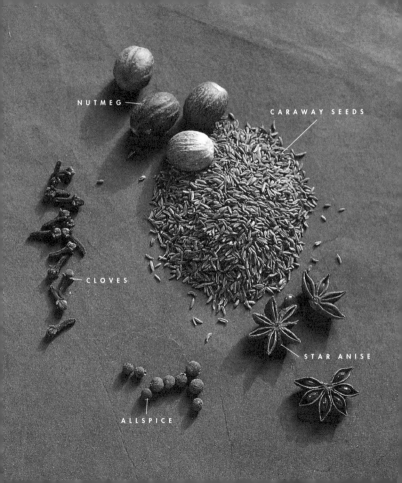

NUTMEG

CARAWAY SEEDS

CLOVES

STAR ANISE

ALLSPICE

Scent Composition. Whether for perfume or potpourri, fragrances are composed using the principle of three "notes" that recognizes the varying intensities and transience of scents and aims to balance them in a lasting bouquet. **TOP NOTES** are the first to strike but are ephemeral. **BASE NOTES**, or "fixatives," provide lasting woody or animal tones that stabilize the entire blend. **MIDDLE NOTES**, typically 50 to 80 percent of the mixture, are the warm heart of the composition. More than one ingredient from each group, particularly of the versatile middle scents, may be used to make a single scent; some perfumes include hundreds. The choices rely on scent-chemistry, personal preference, and intended mood.

> "Stick to simple ideas and
> apply them scrupulously."

PIERRRE FRANÇOIS PASCAL,

perfumer and founder of the House of Guerlain

TOP	BASE	MIDDLE
citrus	balsam	aniseed
clove	benzoin	chamomile
eucalyptus	cedar	cinnamon
marjoram	frankincense	cypress
mint	musk	jasmine
verbena	myrrh	lavender
	oakmoss	melissa
	orrisroot	neroli
	patchouli	rose
	pine	rosemary
	sandalwood	thyme
	storax	
	vanilla	
	vetiver	

SCINTILLATING	SLEEPY	SOOTHING	SEXY
carnation	chamomile	cedar	neroli
clove	fir	chamomile	rose
cypress	lavender	citrus	musk
ginger	lemon thyme	fir	myrrh
juniper	oakmoss	lavender	
marjoram	pine	oakmoss	
mint	rosemary	pine	
nutmeg	vanilla	rose	
rosemary			
thyme			

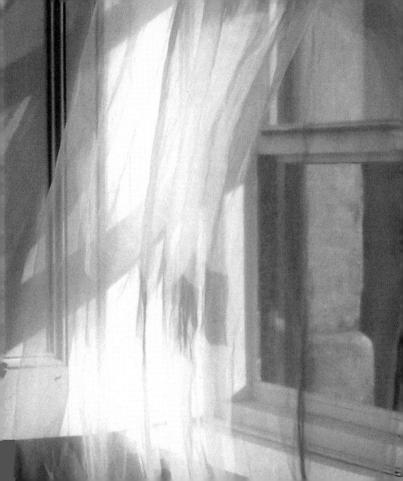

D I F F U S I O N

A breeze, heat, moisture—these are the carriers of scent,
and all means of aromatic diffusion rely on them. Some
methods are as newfangled as microwave potpourri.
Others are as outmoded as the perfumed doves that flew
over galas at Versailles. And some are tried and true.

"The best of our memory lies . . . in
the fragrance of a sealed room or the smell
of something burning."

MARCEL PROUST, *Remembrance of Things Past*

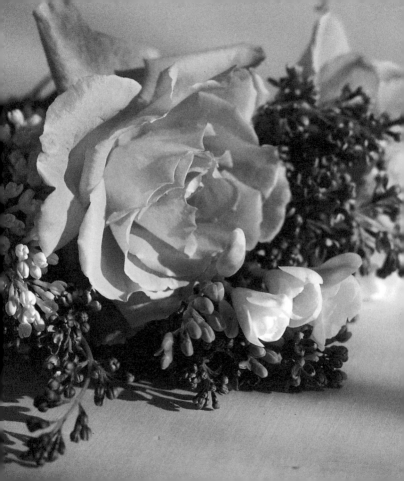

Fresh Bouquets. Floral bouquets, fresh bundles of herbs, and fragrant branches are the most natural way to scent the home. Flowers should be cut from the garden while still dewy, for the rising sun will evaporate up to 20 percent of the essential oil from the petals. Some flowers, such as lilac, madonna lily, narcissus, and tuberose, give off such heady scents that they are best used in large rooms or in a mixed bouquet. Others, particularly roses, have such a balanced scent that they can be used alone. Given the seasonality of fresh botanicals, most homes come to rely on dry or liquid fragrance.

FRENCH COURTS

At the court of Versailles, a special pavilion was filled daily with fresh flowers for Louis XIV to enjoy.

LONDON COURTS

At the criminal courts in London, judges are sometimes presented with floral bouquets and the tables are strewn with herbs, a tradition begun to counteract the disagreeable odors of prisoners.

MIDDLE EASTERN COURTS

The enclosed courtyards of homes in the Middle East are planted with flowers to waft perfume through adjacent chambers.

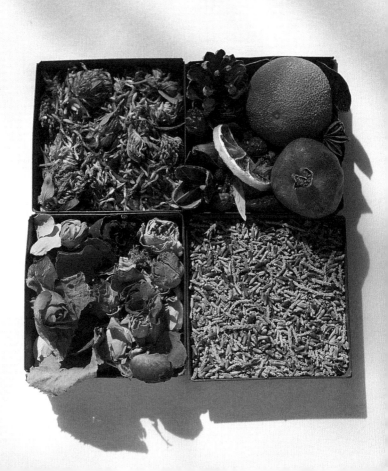

Potpourri. The custom of arranging dried aromatics in an attractive container dates to eighteenth-century Europe. Today's potpourri is often a blend of flowers, leaves, herbs, spices, and fixatives that are all crackling dry (or the mix will mildew), with one or two drops of essential oil added, since most flowers, except the rose, do not retain their scent when dried. The mixture is left to cure for two weeks in a closed paper bag, with an occasional stir, before it is released to diffuse its bouquet from an open bowl placed at some warm or breezy station. If well made, a potpourri will last fifty years.

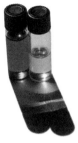

ESSENTIAL OILS
This fragrant extract is highly concentrated— 12,000 pounds of jasmine, for instance, yields two pounds of oil. For most scent purposes, less costly synthetic or adulterated oils can be substituted.

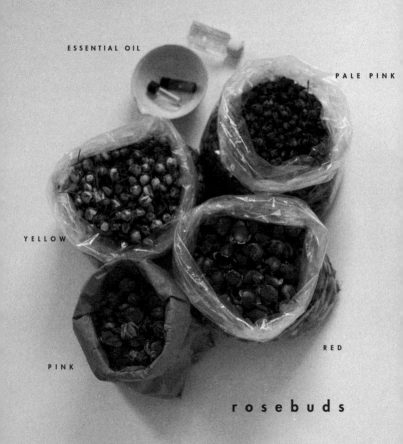

ESSENTIAL OIL

PALE PINK

YELLOW

PINK

RED

rosebuds

LAVENDER

PANSY

XERANTHENUM

MARIGOLD

HEATHER

MARIGOLD

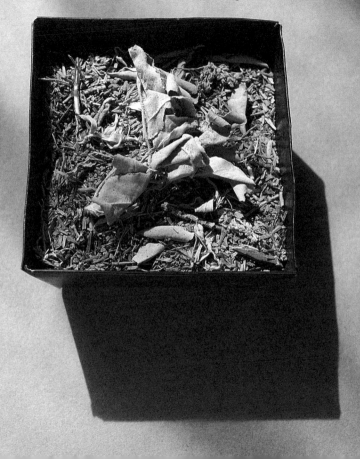

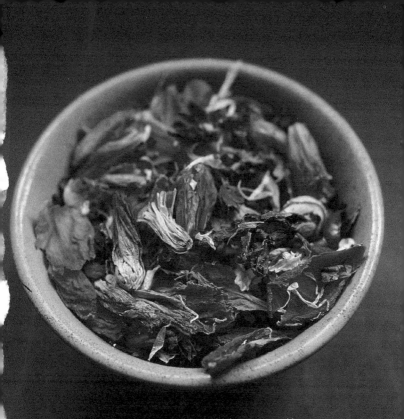

TAMED: peony, hollyhock, delphinium, marigold

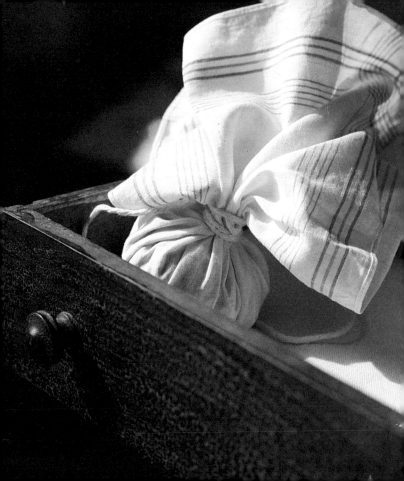

Sachets/Liners. To perfume linens and apparel, sacks made of natural fabrics and filled with potpourri can be tucked into drawers, closets, shoes, and even handbags. Lavender and cedar, nature's own moth repellents, are traditional, but the options for fragrance as well as for shape and placement of sachets are unlimited. In the Middle Ages, people hid herbal packets under seat cushions and doormats, a custom that recognizes the potency of a pressed sachet. A sachet placed in a bed-pillow can release such relaxing aromas as chamomile and vanilla with every movement. As an alternative for scenting drawers, use fabric liners rinsed with rose water or paper liners scented by the same technology as the magazine "scent-strips," which also can be slipped between linens.

ASSORTED STUFFINGS

Romans stuffed their mattresses with rose petals.
Dried leaves of woodruff were placed between book pages in Georgian England.
The poet Schiller kept a desk drawer full of overripe apples.
George III couldn't sleep without his pillow stuffed with hops.

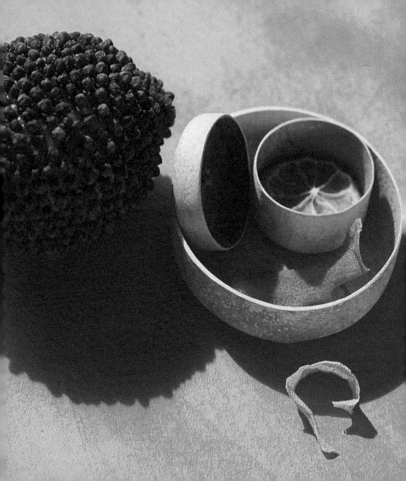

Pomanders. Designed to ward off plague in the seventeenth century, traditional pomanders are of two sorts. The most common one then and now is a dried orange studded with cloves. The grander version is a perforated globe of china or silver filled with aromatics and used in lieu of sachets or potpourri. Some pomanders are especially suitable for moist potpourri, a more potent but visually unattractive cousin to the dry blend. Contemporary additions to the pomander line include boxes and decorative objects fashioned of natural materials, such as citrus rind, or of fragrance-imbued paraffins and woods.

PET POMANDERS

Elizabethan ladies wore their prized pomanders on chains clasped around the neck or girdle when they went out and carried little dogs perfumed to match. When at home, they hung up the pomanders and let the dogs loose to scent their rooms.

STONED POMANDERS

Ground precious stones were sometimes added to pomander mixtures in the seventeenth century.

CLOVE POWER
antiseptic
anesthetic
fungicidal
corrosive

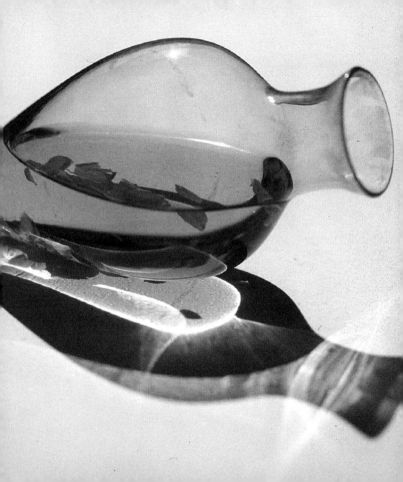

Waters/Sprays. Whether by steam, spray, or slow evaporation, water diffuses scent more effectively than dry ingredients. Aromatics simmered on the stove or radiator have an immediate effect; afterward, the liquid can be strained, cooled, and put out in open flasks for a lasting fragrance. Or, cool water can be scented with drops of essential oil dissolved in alcohol (vodka will do). In lieu of commercial products such as "aerosol deodorizers," use perfume-spritzers to diffuse homemade waters or try the new, more ecologically pleasing pump sprays of natural extracts. It's all in the spritz.

COOLING SYSTEMS
Spray lowers room temperature by displacing heat particles.

A CURTAIN OF SCENT
In India, sun-blinds imbued with vetiver are watered down at midday to add scent to every incoming breeze.

WHOOPIE SPRAY
Romans installed tiny pipes under dinner plates to spritz guests with rose water between courses.

WHOOPIE PART DEUX
Regency women wore "fountain rings" to spritz lovers with perfume as they bent to kiss their hands.

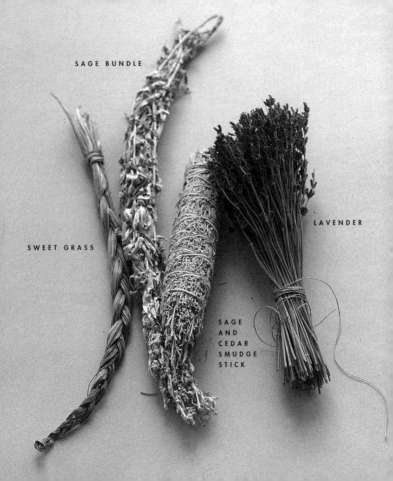

SAGE BUNDLE

SWEET GRASS

SAGE
AND
CEDAR
SMUDGE
STICK

LAVENDER

Wands/Lamps. Smoke-borne fragrance has been popular ever since early man first burned scented wood for perfume. Tightly bound aromatic bundles, or "wands," may be tossed into the fireplace or they may be lit, blown gently, and left to smolder in a ceramic dish. (Before kindling, they might serve as sachets.) Fragrance burners, once pomander-like balls filled with burning incense, are today crafted as capped lamps with wicks partly immersed in liquid perfume; the wick is briefly lit and then extinguished to let the incandescent cap diffuse scent. These smoky aromatics help to bring indoors the primal memories of the outdoors.

TURNED ON
Lamp rings are disks or "moats" resting on light bulbs and dabbed with fragrant oil. Oil can also be applied directly to a cool bulb before it's switched on.

TUNED IN
Cartridges filled with fragrant gels are plugged into outlets; these will soon have "volume" controls to regulate scent.

WIND DOWN
At the entrance of many Arab homes, a charcoal brazier burns incense and wood; arriving guests wrap their cloaks around the brazier for a few minutes to become suffused with the perfume.

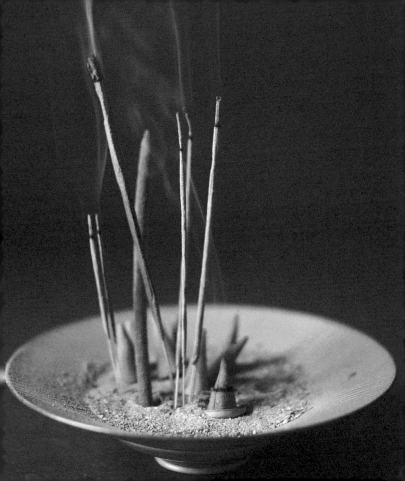

Incense. For at least 4,000 years, incense has been burned through-out the world to perfume homes and religious temples. At his wife Poppaea's funeral, Nero burned more incense than Arabia could pro-duce in one year. In the Eastern tradition, sticks, cones, and tablets are fashioned from blends of sandalwood, gums, and sometimes charcoal, with botanical powders. These are placed in fireproof dishes to burn slowly. The Western tradition holds to the ancient way of burning aro-matics—particularly frankincense and myrrh—over glowing charcoal placed in a brass ornament or "thurible." The Sixties' hippie embraced this ritual by inviting the hallucinatory powers of incense home.

"Incense perfumes bad smells, and candles illumine men's hearts."

CONFUCIUS

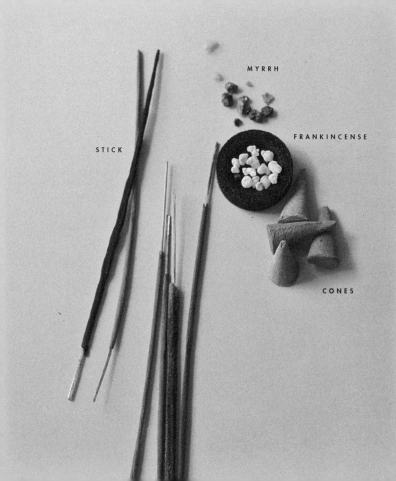

MYRRH

STICK

FRANKINCENSE

CONES

STICKS

*Guessing the kind of incense
and relating it to literary themes
has been a refined "parlor
game" in Japan since the eighth
century, known as Kodo.*

TABLETS

**CRUSHED
INCENSE**

Scented candles are an early Christian tradition and one that gained wider secular favor. Many prefer candles to incense because they are less smoky, although, unless of high quality, they are also less fragrant.

"And sweet's the air with curly smoke
From all my burning bridges."

DOROTHY PARKER

first aid.

Scents, by nature, are organic and temporal; they slip away like all wild things unless they are domesticated. The taming of environmental scent is a function of preservation, storage, rejuvenation, and recycling techniques. The following are tips to keep scent full and fresh throughout the home.

FRESH FLOWERS

Cut at dawn before fragrance evaporates.

To extend life: add a little chlorine bleach and sugar to tepid water; trim stems and change water daily.

To add scent, dab essential oil on greenery.

THE STILL ROOM

The place to dry and store botanicals should be dark and dry and have good air circulation— a closet, cupboard shelf, attic, shed, even under the bed.

DRYING FLOWERS/HERBS

Cut when dry and not overripe at midday.

"Hang dry" long-stem botanicals upside-down in the still room for about a week.

"Air dry" petals and leaves by spreading in a single layer over a flat screen placed in the still room for about a week. Or put the screen in the oven at low heat for about an hour.

For truer flower color and shape, dry with silica gel, a sandlike substance that absorbs vegetal moisture. Gently press flower heads, face up, into a layer of gel, drizzle more gel to completely bury, and cover tightly for a few days—two for a rose, up to seven for fleshier petals and leaves. Remove with slotted spoon.

STORING DRY INGREDIENTS

Place fragrant ingredients, including spices, in airtight glass or ceramic jars in the still room.

Nonfragrant ingredients can be stored in closed paper bags or boxes in the still room.

REFRESHING POTPOURRI / SACHETS

Add essential oil.

Add more ingredients, the same or complementary. A pine cone or dried citrus rind dabbed with oil can add a seasonal touch.

Heat and stir over a light bulb, or heat in a microwave.

Squeeze and scrunch. As for most dry and fresh botanicals, "You must bruise it a little: it does not exude; it yields" (Edna St. Vincent Millay).

LEFTOVER POTPOURRI/SACHETS

Toss into fireplace.

Simmer in water on the stove.

Use sachets in bath or shower.

MOIST POTPOURRI

Make a moist potpourri by mixing five parts semidry ingredients layered with one part salt and fermenting for two months.

ESSENTIAL OILS

Kept away from light and air, essential oils will last three years.

Many are toxic, even fatal, if ingested; do not use as flavorings.

Essential oils will stain like any oil; don't put on clothing.

LEFTOVER USES

Dab on heat sources such as light bulbs (when cool), radiators, sauna braziers, or on absorbent materials such as the underside of wooden furniture or window blinds.

Blend with "carrier oils" such as almond, soy, or jojoba and use in your bath or for aromatherapy massage. Always do a skin test first, for some oils can be irritating; dab blend on inside area of one elbow and wait for 24 hours to see if there's any adverse reaction. Store in the refrigerator and they'll keep at least six months.

POMANDERS: HOW TO

Make a clove-studded orange last forever by turning it regularly in a mix of powdered spice and fixatives over several weeks until it has hardened.

ROSE WATER: HOW TO

"Mix rose-oil drops into a cup of water, then one drop at a time, add a solubilizer (available in the cosmetics sections of natural-food stores) to make the oil and water mix. Set petals afloat, but change them regularly, since they turn brown within a few days."–Martha Stewart Living, *June–July 1993*

THE EIGHT PERSONALITIES OF PERFUME

Single florals, such as rose or jasmine

Floral bouquets: a blend with base notes of woods and greens

Spicy notes such as carnation and lavender

Woodsy-mossy: fragrances heavy with aromatic woods—particularly sandalwood, rosewood, and cedar—combined with oakmoss and fern

Oriental: sultry blends of animal scents with exotic flowers, woods, resins, and spice

Fruity: a mix of florals topped by a citrus freshness

Green: compositions with a high note of herbs or coumarin (the scent of fresh-cut hay)

Aldehydic: perfumes that include an organic chemical, derived from natural material or produced synthetically, which lend lasting richness to fragrance warmed on the skin

CANDLES

Waxes: Beeswax exudes a honey scent and burns slowly; paraffin is naturally odorless; stearin is mixed with paraffin to prevent dripping.

Candles are scented by stirring dried herbs or special oils in the melted wax before molding.

Candle scent can be revived by a drop of scented oil to the well beneath the wick.

Flattop candles do not burn as effectively as pointed ones.

INCENSE

Instant incense: Light a nut of barbecue charcoal in an incense burner and, after the flame has died to a gentle smolder, sprinkle with two teaspoons of dried herbs and spices.

Always ventilate a room where incense is burned, as charcoal fumes can be harmful.

where.

A Chic Simple store looks out on the world beyond its shop window. Items are practical and comfortable and will work with pieces bought elsewhere. The store can be a cottage industry or a global chain but even with an international vision it is still rooted in tradition, quality, and value.

United States

ARIZONA

CRYSTAL CASTLE
313 Highway 179
Sedona, AZ 86336
602/282-5910
(Aromatherapy and scented oils)

ARKANSAS

AROMATIQUE, INC.
3421 Highway 25 North
Heber Springs, AR 72543
501/362-7511
(Manufacturer of decorative room fragrance composed of dried botanicals; factory store)

CALIFORNIA

FILLAMENTO
2185 Fillmore Street
San Francisco, CA 94115
415/931-2224
(Scented soaps)

FRED SEGAL
ENVIRONMENT
420 Broadway
Santa Monica, CA 90401
310/394-7088
(Aromatherapy, essential oils)

FRED SEGAL
SCENTIMENTS
500 Broadway
Santa Monica, CA 90401
310/394-8509
(Scented candles, lotions, body oils)

MOTHER'S MARKET
225 East 17th Street
Costa Mesa, CA 92627
714/631-4741
(Essential oils, aromatherapy)

PALMETTO
1034 Montana Avenue
Santa Monica, CA 90403
310/395-6687
(Scented bath oils)

SKIN ZONE
575 Castro Street
San Francisco, CA 94114
415/626-7933
(Scented bath oils, colognes)

SWEET IVY
3470 Blackhawk Plaza Circle
Danville, CA 94506
510/736-0949
(Potpourri, scented candles)

COLORADO

ALFALFA'S MARKET
1645 Broadway
Boulder, CO 80302
303/442-0909 for statewide
listings
(Fresh and dry botanicals)

FLORIDA

BEACH NEWS
651 Washington Avenue
Miami Beach, FL 33139
305/672-0081
(Incense, candles)

BURDINES
1675 Meridian Ave.
Miami Beach, FL 33139
305/835-5151
Catalogue available
(Fragrances)

FAST BUCK FREDDIE'S
500 Duval Street
Key West, FL 33040
305/294-2007
*(Aromatherapy, scented
candles, potpourri)*

GEORGIA

HOSPITALITY HOUSE
2359 Peachtree Road, N.E.
Atlanta, GA 30305
404/237-1119
(Scented lotions, oils, candles)

RICH'S
Lenox Square Shopping Mall
3393 Peachtree Road
Atlanta, GA 30326
404/231-2611
(Fragrances, scented lotions)

HAWAII

LIBERTY HOUSE
Ala Moana
Waikiki Beach
Honolulu, HI 96845
808/941-2345
(Fragrance department)

ILLINOIS

ELEMENTS
738 North Wells Street
Chicago, IL 60610
312/642-6574
(Potpourri, sachet pillows)

GOOD SCENTS
330 Old McHenry Road
Long Grove, IL 60047
708/634-2010
*(Candles, oils, potpourri,
incense)*

IMPULSE
261 East Market Square
Lake Forest, IL 60045
708/234-0709
(Bath soaps, oils)

LOUISIANA

BELLADONNA
1720 St. Charles Avenue
New Orleans, LA 70130
504/581-6759
*(Potpourri, scented candles
and oils, herbal baths)*

MINNESOTA

PRESENT MOMENT
3546 Grand Avenue South
Minneapolis, MN 55408
612/824-3157
(Essential oils, aromatherapy)

NEW MEXICO

WILD OATS MARKET
1090 South St. Francis Drive
Santa Fe, NM 87501
505/983-5333
*(Herbs, dried flowers,
aromatherapy, essential oils)*

NEW YORK

ABC CARPET & HOME
BATH, BED & LINEN
SHOP
888 Broadway
New York, NY 10003
212/473-3000
(Scented candles)

AD HOC SOFTWARES
410 West Broadway
New York, NY 10012
212/925-2652
(Scented candles)

ANGELICA'S
147 First Avenue
New York, NY 10003
212/677-1549
(Traditional herbs and spices)

AVEDA ESTHETIQUE
509 Madison Avenue
New York, NY 10022
212/832-2416
(Scented oils)

AYURVEDA
129 First Avenue
New York, NY 10003
212/260-1218
*(Herbal extracts, oils,
shampoos, essential oils,
aromatherapy baths)*

BATH & BODY WORKS
89 South Street
Pier 17
New York, NY 10038
212/693-0247
*(Scented candles, books on
how to create a scented room,
such as The Scented Room
from Clarkson Potter)*

BATH ISLAND
469 Amsterdam Avenue
New York, NY 10024
212/787-9415
(Scented oils, soaps)

BERGDORF GOODMAN
754 Fifth Avenue
New York, NY 10019
212/753-7300
(Fragrance department)

CAMBRIDGE CHEMISTS
21 East 65th Street
New York, NY 10021
212/734-5678
(Scented candles, potpourri)

DEAN & DELUCA
560 Broadway
New York, NY 10012
212/431-1691
*(Scented body oils, fresh
flowers)*

FELISSIMO
10 West 56th Street
New York, NY 10019
212/956-4438
*(Environmentally safe room
sprays, aromatherapy oils)*

FLORIS OF LONDON
703 Madison Avenue
New York, NY 10021
212/935-9100
*(Fragrances, bath products,
and accessories)*

GABAY'S OUTLET
225 First Avenue
New York, NY 10003
212/254-3180
(Assorted scent products)

GALERIES LAFAYETTE
10 East 57th Street
New York, NY 10022
212/355-0022
(Fragrance department)

JANOVIC/PLAZA
1150 Third Avenue
New York, NY 10021
212/772-1400 for info and
other Manhattan locations
(Potpourri, scented soaps)

KIEHL'S
109 Third Avenue
New York, NY 10019
212/677-3171
(Scented lotions, fragrances)

L'ARTISAN
PARFUMEUR
870 Madison Avenue
New York, NY 10021
212/517-8665
(*Fragrances*)

LORD & TAYLOR
424 Fifth Avenue
New York, NY 10018
212/391-3344
(*Fragrance department*)

MARDERS NURSERIES
P.O. Box 1261
Bridgehampton, NY 11932
516/537-3700
(*Ships plants nationwide*)

MATTERHORN
NURSERY
227 Summit Park Road
Spring Valley, NY 10977
914/354-5986
Catalogue and newsletter
available
(*Ornamental grasses, hostas,
ferns, and waterplants*)

MUSEUM OF AMERICAN
FOLK ART BOOK AND
GIFT SHOP
62 West 50th Street
New York, NY 10112
212/247-5611

2 Lincoln Square
New York, NY 10023
212/496-2966
(*Scented soaps*)

PAUL BOTT
BEAUTIFUL FLOWERS
1305 Madison Avenue
New York, NY 10128
212/369-4000
(*Cut flowers, potpourri,
topiary*)

SAKS FIFTH AVENUE
611 Fifth Avenue
New York, NY 10022
212/753-4000 for U.S.
listings
(*Assorted scent products*)

SEASONS, A FLORAL
DESIGN STUDIO
888 Eighth Avenue
New York, NY 10019
212/586-2257
(*Unusual plants, baskets,
pottery*)

TERRA VERDE
TRADING CO.
120 Wooster Street
New York, NY 10012
212/925-4533
(*Cedar chips and oil*)

WOLFMAN•GOLD &
GOOD COMPANY
116 Greene Street
New York, NY 10012
212/431-1888
(*Dried fruit, flowers and
herbs, room sprays, potpourri*)

SOUTH DAKOTA

STAPLE AND SPICE
MARKET
601 Mt. Rushmore Road
Rapid City, SD 57701
605/343-3900
(*Bulk herbs and spices*)

VERMONT

SEVENTH GENERATION
49 Hercules Drive
Colchester, VT 05446-1672
802/655-6777

176 Battery Street
Burlington, VT 05401
802/658-7770
800/456-1177 mail and
telephone orders
(*Soaps and body creams*)

WASHINGTON

ZANADIA
1815 North 45th Street
Space 218
Seattle, WA 98103
206/547-0884
*(Scented acorns, room sprays,
perfumed candles)*

WISCONSIN

CAROLINA DESIGNS
FACTORY OUTLET
Oshkosh, WI 54901
414/233-3214
*(Microwave potpourri,
candles)*

NATIONAL AND
INTERNATIONAL
LISTINGS

BARNEYS NEW YORK
Apothecary Department,
main floor
111 Seventh Avenue
New York, NY 10011
212/929-9000
800/777-0087
*(Candles, fragrances, essential
oils)*

BED BATH & BEYOND
620 Avenue of the Americas
New York, NY 10011
212/255-3550
(Scented candles)

HENRI BENDEL
712 Fifth Avenue
New York, NY 10019
212/247-1100
(Fragrances, scented lotions)

BLOOMINGDALE'S
1000 Third Avenue
New York, NY 10022
212/355-5900 for U.S.
listings
(Fragrance department)

THE BODY SHOP
45 Horsehill Road
Cedar Knolls, NJ 07927
800/541-2535 for U.S. listings
903/731-500 for U.K. listings
(Potpourri, scented soaps, oils)

CASWELL-MASSEY
518 Lexington Avenue
New York, NY 10017
212/755-2254
800/326-0500 for other
store locations
*(Dried herbs, potpourri, sachet
pillows, colognes)*

CRABTREE & EVELYN
1310 Madison Avenue
New York, NY 10128
212/289-3923
800/624-5211 for U.S.
listings
*(Fragrances, room sprays,
environmental oils, potpourri)*

DAYTON HUDSON CORP.
(DAYTON'S, HUDSON'S,
MARSHALL FIELD'S)
700 On The Mall
Minneapolis, MN 55402
612/375-2200 for U.S.
listings
(Fragrance department)

DESCAMPS
723 Madison Avenue
New York, NY 10021
212/355-2522
(Scented and herbal soaps)

DILLARD'S PARK PLAZA
Markham & University
Little Rock, AR 72205
501/661-0053
(Fragrances)

EMPORIO ARMANI
110 Fifth Avenue
New York, NY 10011
212/727-3240
Catalogue available
(Scented soaps)

GARDEN BOTANIKA
Washington Square Mall
9508 SW Washington
Square Boulevard
Tigard, OR 97223
503/620-1975
800/877-9603 for West
Coast listings
*(Custom-scented bath
products)*

GEORGETTE KLINGER
501 Madison Avenue
New York, NY 10022
212/838-3200
800/KLINGER outside New
York City
(Herbal body lotions and bath
refresheners, scented
moisturizers, hand soaps,
candles)

GOODEBODIES
Cocowalk
3015 Grand Avenue
Coconut Grove, FL 33133
305/444-8350
800/966-3993 for mail
order and U.S. listings
(Essential and scented oils,
potpourri, scented candles,
fragrances)

HOLD EVERYTHING
P.O. Box 7807
San Francisco, CA 94120
800/421-2264 for mail
order catalogue and store
locations
(Bathroom accessories)

HOME DEPOT
449 Roberts Court Road
Kennesaw, GA 30144
404/433-8211
(Bath accessories)

IKEA
1000 Town Center Drive
Elizabeth, NJ 07201
908/289-4488
412/747-0747 for East Coast
listings
818/842-4532 for West
Coast listings
Catalogue available
(Live plants and flowers)

R.H. MACY INC.
(BULLOCK'S, I. MAGNIN,
AÉROPOSTALE)
MACY'S HERALD SQUARE
151 West 34th Street
New York, NY 10001
212/695-4400 for East Coast
listings
415/393-3457 for West
Coast listings
(Fragrances, potpourri)

MAY D & F
(FOLEY'S,
ROBINSON'S, MAY)
16th at Tremont Place
Denver, CO 80202
(303)620-9005 for U.S.
listings
(Fragrance department)

NATURE'S ELEMENTS
115 River Road
Edgewater, NJ 07020
800/545-1325 for MA, NJ,
NY, PA, and VT stores
Catalogue available
(Sachets, potpourri, scented
beads, fragrance sprays,
candles)

NEIMAN MARCUS
1618 Main Street
Dallas, TX 75201
210/573-5780
(Fragrance department)

NORDSTROM
1501 Fifth Avenue
Seattle, WA 98191
206/628-2111
800/285-5800 for
Nordstrom catalogue
(Fragrance department)

ORIGINS
402 West Broadway
New York, NY 10012
212/219-9764
800/ORIGINS for U.S.
listings
(Skin care, sensory therapy oils
and gels)

PARISIAN
2100 River Chase Galleria
Birmingham, AL 35244
(205) 987-4200
(205) 940-4000 for U.S.
listings
(Fragrance department)

PIER 1 IMPORTS
P.O. Box 961020
Ft. Worth, TX 76161
800/447-4371
*(Room sprays, fresheners,
scented soaps)*

POLO/RALPH LAUREN
HOME COLLECTION
867 Madison Avenue
New York, NY 10021
212/606-2100
*(Scented candles, room sprays,
potpourri, sachets)*

URBAN OUTFITTERS
4040 Locust Street
Philadelphia, PA 19104
215/569-3131
215/564-2313 for U.S.
listings
(Incense, potpourri)

ZONA
97 Greene Street
New York, NY 10012
212/925-6750
(Dried flowers, potpourri)

CATALOGUES AND
MAIL ORDER

AGRARIA
1051 Howard Street
San Francisco, CA 94103
800/824-3632
(Scented soaps, potpourri)

AVON
800/FOR-AVON
(Fragrances, scented lotions)

BASICALLY NATURAL
109 East G Street
Brunswick, MD 21716
301/834-7923
(Herbal hair care)

THE COMPASSIONATE
CONSUMER
P.O. Box 27
Jericho, NY 11753
718/445-4134
(Cruelty-free perfumes)

ECCO BELLA
125 Pompton Plains
Crossroad
Wayne, NJ 07470
800/322-9344
*(Cruelty-free massage oils and
perfumes)*

FIGIS
3200 South Maple Avenue
Marshfield, WI 54449
715/384-6101
(Fresh and dried flowers)

GARDENERS EDEN
P.O. Box 7307
San Francisco, CA 94133
800/822-9600
*(Flowering plants and
wreaths)*

HARRY AND DAVID
2518 South Pacific Highway
Medford, OR 97501
800/547-3033
(Decorative plants)

HUMANE
ALTERNATIVE
PRODUCTS
8 Hutchins Street
Concord, NH 03301
603/224-1361
*(Cruelty-free perfumes and
colognes)*

LITTLE RED'S WORLD
720 Greenwich Street
Suite 7K
New York, NY 10014
212/807-0452
*(Environmentally friendly
personal-care products)*

NATIONAL WILDLIFE
NATURE GIFTS
National Wildlife
Federation
1400 Sixteenth Street, N.W.
Washington, DC 20036
800/432-6564
(Scented stationery, citronella candles)

ORCHIDS ONLY
1 Orchid Lane
Medford, OR 97501
800/423-2806
(Blooming plants, floral bouquets, tropical orchid baskets)

YVES ROCHER
301 Brandywine Parkway
West Chester, PA 19380
800/321-9837
(Fragrances and related products)

INTERNATIONAL LISTINGS

Australia

MELBOURNE

GEORGES AUSTRALIA, LIMITED
162 Collins Street
Melbourne 3000
3/283-5555
(Fragrance department)

SYDNEY

GRACE BROS.
436 George Street
NSW 2000
2/238-9111
(Scented bath oils and lotions)

THE MAGIC GUMNUT
Shop 487, Harbourside
Darling Harbour, NSW 2000
2/281-4345
(Aromatherapy, potpourri, scented candles, and bath products)

REMO CITY VENTURES
82 Oxford Street
Darlinghurst, NSW 2010
2/331-5544
Catalogue available

Canada

MONTREAL

EATON
677 Ste-Catherine Ouest
514/284-8484
(Fragrance department)

OGILVY
1307 Ste-Catherine Ouest
514/842-7711
(Perfumed soaps and lotions in fragrance department)

ST. JACQUES MARKET
1125 Ontario East Street
514/872-2491
(Market with flowers and plants; open May–October)

QUEBEC

PUR ET SIMPLE
Ayers Cliff
Quebec City
418/522-3645
(Soaps, lotions, herbal baths)

TORONTO

ALFRED SUNG
Hazelton Lanes
87 Avenue Road M5R 3L2
416/922-9226
(Fragrances, scented lotions)

HOLT RENFREW
50 Bloor Street West
416/922-2333 for Canadian listings
(Fragrances, sachet pillows, potpourri)

France

ANNICK GOUTAL
259, rue St. Honoré
75001
45/51-36-13 for Paris
listings
*(Fragrances, perfumes, and
perfumed products)*

GALERIES LAFAYETTE
40 boulevard Haussmann
75009
42/82-34-56
(Fragrance department)

GUERLAIN
68, avenue des Champs-
Elysées
75008
47/89-71-84 for Paris
listings
*(Perfumes and perfumed
products)*

L'HERBIER DE
PROVENCE
Forum des Halles, Level 2
42/97-46-44
*(Potpourri, candles, scented
soaps)*

HERBORISTERIE DE LA
PLACE CLICHY
87, rue d'Amsterdam
75008
48/74-83-32
*(Herbs, essential oils, rose
water)*

HERBORISTERIE DU
PALAIS-ROYAL
11, rue des Petits-Champs
75001
42/97-54-68
*(Aromatic plants and
medicines)*

INTERFLORA
05/20-32-04 toll free in
France; U.S. customers
contact local florist
(Flowers by phone)

JULE DES PRÈS
19, rue du Cherche-Midi
75006
45/48-26-84
(Dried herbs and flowers)

LACHAUME
10, rue Royale
75008
42/60-59-74
(Flowers)

LE SORBIER DES
OISELEURS
70, rue Vieille-du-Temple
75003
48/87-69-72
(Dried flowers)

LILIANE FRANÇOIS
119, rue de Grenelle
75007
45/51-73-18

64, rue de Longchamp
75016
47/27-51-52
(Dried and fresh flowers)

PARFUM CARON
34, avenue Montaigne
75008
47/23-40-82
(Perfumes, perfume bottles)

PIERRE DECLERCQ
83, avenue Kleber
75016
45/43-45-56
(Florist)

PRINTEMPS
64, boulevard Haussmann
75009
42/82-50-00
(Fragrance department)

ROCHAS
33, rue François
75001
47/23-54-56
(Fragrances, scent products)

Germany

BERLIN

SELBACH
Kurfürstendamm 195/196
1000 Berlin 15
30/883-2526
(Fragrance department)

FRANKFURT

PARFUMERIE DOUGLAS
69/28-79-12 for information
and 10 Frankfurt locations

MUNICH

MEY & EDLICH
Theatinerstrasse 7
80333
89/290-0590 for store
locations
*(Fragrances, potpourri,
sachets)*

Great Britain

CAMBRIDGE

CULPEPER LTD.
Hadstock Road
Linton, CB1 6NJ
223/894-054 for U.K.
listings
*(Mail-order potted and dried
herbs, sachets, potpourri)*

LONDON

CRABTREE & EVELYN
55-57 South Edwardes
Square
W8 6HP
071/603-1611

CULPEPER THE
HERBALISTS
21 Bruton Street,
Berkeley Square
W1X 7DA
071/629-4559

COSMETICS TO GO
Poole
Dorset, BH15 1BR
800/373-366
Mail-order service
(Bath products)

CZECH AND SPEAKE
LTD.
244-254 Cambridge Heath
Road
E2 9DA
81/980-4567
*(Potpourri, scented oils,
colognes)*

FLORIS PERFUMERS
89 Jermyn Street
SW1Y 6JH
71/930-2885
(Scents and toilet waters)

THE GENERAL
TRADING COMPANY
144 Sloan Square
SW1X 9BL
071/930-0411

GEO F. TRUMPER
9 Curzon Street
Mayfair
W1Y 7FL
71/499-1850
*(Gentlemen's hairdresser and
perfumer)*

HACKETTS
136-138 Sloan Street
SW1
071/730-3331

HARRODS, LIMITED
87-135 Brompton Road
Knightsbridge
SW1X 7XL
71/730-1234
(Fragrances, potpourri,
sachets)

HEALS
196 Tottenham Court Road
W1A 1BJ
071/636-1666

LIBERTY, PLC
The Bath House
210-220 Regent Street
W1R 6AH
71/734-1234
(Fragrances, potpourri,
sachets)

MARKS & SPENCER
113 Kensington High Street
W8 5SQ
71/938-3711
(Assortment of scented
personal-care products)

NEAL'S YARD REMEDIES
1A Rossiter Road
Balham
SW12 9RY
81/675-7144
Mail-order service
(Aromatic oils, flower
remedies, herbs, skin oils)

PENHALIGON'S
PERFUMERS LTD.
41 Wellington Street
WC2E 7BN
71/836-2150
81/880-2050 for mail order
(Old-fashioned English scents
and scent bottles)

SELFRIDGES
400 Oxford Street
W1A 1AB
71/629-1234
(Largest perfumery in Europe)

SUFFOLK

CULPEPER HERB
GARDEN
44/085-228 to arrange a
visit

Italy

FLORENCE

OFFICINA PROFUMO
FARMACEUTICA DI
SANTA MARIA
NOVELLA
via della Scala, 16
50123
55/21-62-76
(Potpourri, herbs, room
fragrances)

MILAN

DUOMO FLOWER
MARKET
Piazzetta Reale
(Flowers and plants; Sunday
mornings)

ERBORISTERIA
MILANO
via Montegarni, 20
20142
2/89-50-11-52
(Herbs, perfumed soaps)

ROME

ERBORISTERIA IL
SOLE E LA TERRA
via Pietro Bembo, 14
00168
6/35-50-39-50
(Herbs, potpourri, sachets)

Japan

TOKYO

AQUAPLA
3-7-2 Jiyugaoka
Meguro-ku
3/3725-5277
(Scented bathing products)

ISETAN
3-14-1 Shinjuku-ku
3/3352-1111
(Fragrance department,
potpourri, sachets)

MITSUKOSHI
1-4-1 Nihonbashi
Muromachi
Chuo-ku
3/3241-3311
(Fragrance department)

MUJIRUSHI
5-50-6 Jingumae
Shibuya-ku
3/3407-4666
*(No-name-brand scented
lotions, oils)*

PARCO I, II, III
14 Udagawa-cho
Shibuya-ku
3/3464-5111
*(Various boutiques selling
scented products)*

TAKASHIMAYA
4-4-1 Nihonbashi
Chuo-ku
3/3211-4111
(Assorted fragrance products)

TINAMARRY
20-13
Sarugakucho
Shibuya-ku
3/5489-9800
(Scented skincare products)

RESOURCES

COVER FRONT

LILY OF THE VALLEY - S. S. Pennock
Co., New York

BACK

PERFUME BOTTLES - Barneys New York

SCENTS

14 **BASEBALL MITT** - from the private
collection of Bradley Friedman
19 (From top left): **CUP & SAUCER** -
Wolfman • Gold & Good Co.;
PERFUME BOTTLES - Barneys New York;
GLASS POT - Gracious Home,
New York; **VICKS VAPORUB**
66 **CITRUS BOXES** - Origins, Bergdorf
Goodman, New York
68 **ROSE WATER** - Kiehl's, New York
72 **SCENT BUNDLES** - (from left):
SWEET GRASS - Common Ground,
New York; **SAGE BUNDLE** - Common
Ground, New York; **SAGE & CEDAR
SMUDGE STICK** - Native Scents, Taos,
New Mexico; **LAVENDER BUNDLE** -
Zona, New York
78–79 **CANDLES** - Ad Hoc Softwares, New York

QUOTES

2   JEAN-JACQUES ROUSSEAU, *Emile* (Paris: Gallimard, 1969)

11   RUDYARD KIPLING, as quoted in *A Natural History of the Senses* by Diane Ackerman (New York: Random House, 1990)

13   EDWARD THOMAS, *The Macmillan Dictionary of Quotations* (1987)

23   MUHAMMAD ALI, ibid.

31   GIORGIO ARMANI, *Perfumes: The Essences and Their Bottles* by Jean-Yves Gaborit (New York: Rizzoli Intl., 1985)

43   GERTRUDE STEIN, *Sacred Emily* (1913)

45   CHANG CHEN, A.D. 725

54   GUERLAIN, *Perfumes: The Essences and Their Bottles* by Jean-Yves Gaborit (New York: Rizzoli Intl., 1985)

57   MARCEL PROUST, *Remembrance of Things Past* (New York: Vintage Books, Random House, 1992)

75   CONFUCIUS, 551-479 B.C.

79   DOROTHY PARKER, "Sanctuary," *The Portable Dorothy Parker* (New York: Viking, 1944)

96   ALBERT EINSTEIN, as quoted in *Scents and Sensuality* by Max Lake (1989)

ACKNOWLEDGMENTS

Rosie Boycott, Beth Chang, Tony Chirico, Lauri Del Commune, M. Scott Cookson, Dina Dell'Arciprete, Chris DiMaggio, Michael Drazen, Felissimo, Marion Fouretier, The Fragrance Foundation, Jane Friedman, Janice Goldklang, Jo-Anne Harrison, Patrick Higgins, Katherine Hourigan, Andy Hughes, Carole Janeway, Nicholas Latimer, Karen Leh, William Loverd, Joel Makower, Anne McCormick, Mary McEvoy, Sonny Mehta, Olfactory Research Fund, Hellyn Sher, Anne-Lise Spitzer, Meg Stebbins, Robin Swados, Kim Turner, Shelley Wanger, Wayne Wolf, Alice Wong.

A NOTE ON THE TYPE

The text of this book was set in New Baskerville, the ITC version of the typeface called Baskerville, which itself is a facsimile reproduction of types cast from molds made by John Baskerville (1706–1775) from his designs. Baskerville's original face was one of the forerunners of the type style known to printers as the "modern face"—a "modern" of the period A.D. 1800.

SEPARATION AND FILM PREPARATION BY
APPLIED GRAPHICS TECHNOLOGIES
Carlstadt, New Jersey

PRINTED AND BOUND BY
BERTELSMANN PRINTING & MANUFACTURING CORP.
Berryville, Virginia

"Everything should be made as simple as possible, but not simpler."

ALBERT EINSTEIN

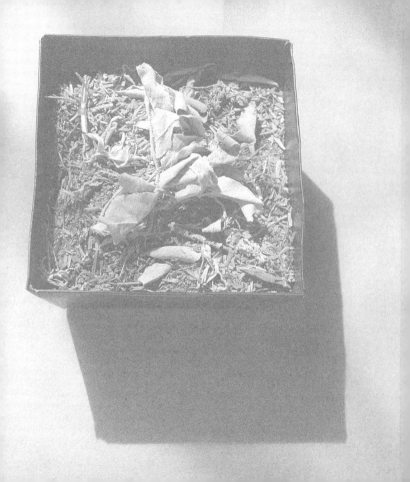